THE MEDITERRANEAN DASH DIET COOKBOOK

62 Stress-Free And Mouth Watery Recipes To Lower Your Blood Pressure And Effortlessly Lose Weight For LifeLong Health

Jennifer J Rodriguez

62 recipes and 28-days meal plans to **kick start your day**

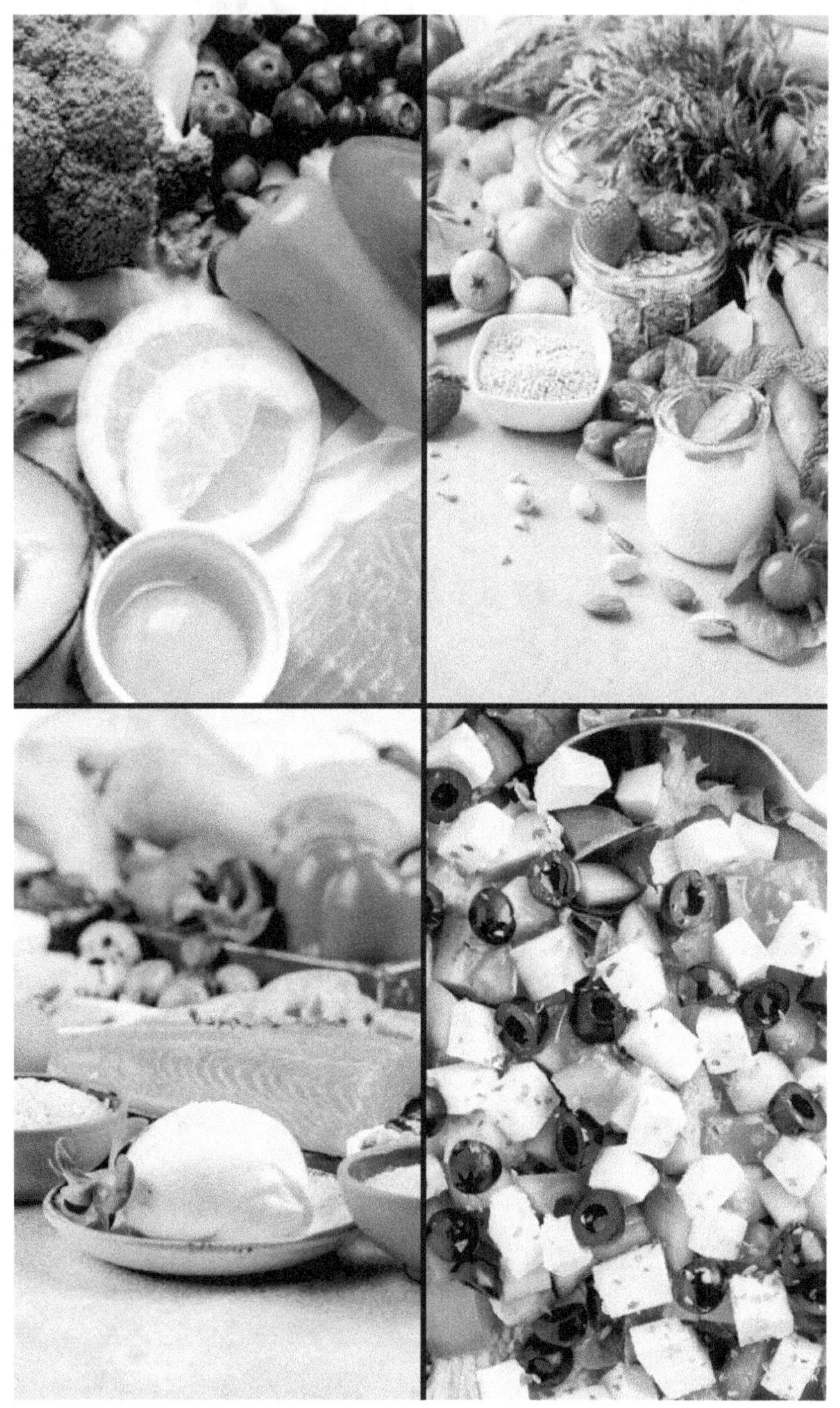

The Mediterranean dash diet cookbook

TABLE OF CONTENT

INTRODUCTION TO THE MEDITERRANEAN DASH DIET

Imagine waking up every morning with a renewed sense of vitality and purpose, feeling the gentle Mediterranean breeze caress your skin as you embark on a journey towards a healthier you. Meet Juliet, a vibrant and determined individual who, despite grappling with the challenges of high blood pressure and fluctuating energy levels, discovered the transformative power of the Mediterranean DASH Diet. With the guidance of this culinary philosophy, she not only regained control over her health but also unearthed a newfound love for nourishing, flavor-packed meals that invigorated her body and soul. Join us as we unravel the secrets behind this life-changing diet and unlock the gateway to a world of vibrant flavors and rejuvenated well-being.

Embracing the Mediterranean DASH Diet: A Flavorful Fusion

In a world brimming with fad diets and fleeting wellness trends, the Mediterranean DASH Diet stands as a beacon of sustainable and holistic nourishment. Rooted in the heart-healthy culinary traditions of the Mediterranean region and fortified by the evidence-based principles of the Dietary Approaches to Stop Hypertension (DASH), this dietary approach intertwines the bounties of fresh produce, lean proteins, and heart-healthy fats to create a harmonious symphony of flavors and wellness. With a focus on balancing nutrient-rich ingredients and minimizing sodium intake, this diet not only fosters cardiovascular health but also promotes overall vitality and longevity.

Unlocking the Essence of the Mediterranean DASH Diet

At its core, the Mediterranean DASH Diet transcends the limitations of a mere meal plan; it embodies a lifestyle brimming with the richness of wholesome ingredients and the joy of communal dining experiences.

Encapsulating the essence of sun-kissed vegetables, succulent seafood, aromatic herbs, and wholesome grains, this diet encourages individuals to savor each bite mindfully and embrace the nourishing bounty of the earth. With an emphasis on incorporating heart-healthy fats, such as olive oil and nuts, alongside a medley of vibrant fruits and vegetables, this diet transcends the boundaries of restriction and welcomes all to relish the abundance of nature's offerings.

A Culinary Adventure Awaits

As you embark on this culinary adventure through the pages of our cookbook, prepare to be tantalized by the tantalizing aromas and exquisite flavors that define the essence of the Mediterranean DASH Diet. From the crispness of freshly harvested salads to the indulgence of delicately spiced seafood, each recipe has been meticulously crafted to not only tantalize your taste buds but also nourish your body from within. Join us as we dive deep into the heart of this enchanting gastronomic journey and discover the transformative power of the Mediterranean DASH Diet—a voyage that promises not only a healthier you but a rekindled love for the art of savoring life's simple pleasures.

Embrace the richness of the Mediterranean DASH Diet and let the flavors of the sun-kissed region guide you towards a life of vitality, wellness, and everlasting culinary bliss.

PART 1: UNDERSTANDING THE BASICS OF THE MEDITERRANEAN DIET

The Mediterranean diet is not just a way of eating but a lifestyle inspired by the traditional dietary patterns of the countries bordering the Mediterranean Sea. It emphasizes the consumption of whole, plant-based foods, lean proteins, and healthy fats, while minimizing the intake of processed and red meats, refined sugars, and saturated fats. This approach is rooted in the abundance of fresh fruits and vegetables, whole grains, legumes, nuts, and olive oil, all of which are fundamental components of the Mediterranean diet.

The diet is characterized by a high consumption of vegetables, fruits, and whole grains, as well as a moderate intake of fish, poultry, and red wine. It promotes the use of herbs and spices to add flavor, rather than relying on salt, and encourages regular physical activity and the enjoyment of meals with family and friends. This dietary pattern has been associated with numerous health benefits, including reduced risks of heart disease, certain cancers, and cognitive decline.

The Principles of the DASH Diet

The Dietary Approaches to Stop Hypertension (DASH) diet was developed to help lower blood pressure without the need for medication. It emphasizes the consumption of fruits, vegetables, whole grains, and lean proteins while limiting the intake of high-fat, high-sodium, and sugary foods. The DASH diet encourages the reduction of sodium intake, which is known to contribute to high blood pressure, and promotes the consumption of foods rich in potassium, calcium, and magnesium, all of which are vital for maintaining healthy blood pressure levels.

This diet is not only effective in managing blood pressure but also aids in weight loss, reducing the risk of heart disease, stroke, and certain types of cancer. The DASH diet encourages individuals to adopt a balanced and nutrient-rich eating pattern that prioritizes whole, unprocessed foods and limits the consumption of saturated fats and added sugars.

The Fusion of the Mediterranean DASH Diet

The fusion of the Mediterranean and DASH diets combines the best of both worlds, creating a powerful dietary approach that promotes overall health and well-being. By integrating the heart-healthy and blood-pressure-lowering aspects of both diets, this fusion emphasizes the consumption of nutrient-dense foods, such as fresh fruits, vegetables, whole grains, lean proteins, and healthy fats, while minimizing the intake of processed and high-sodium foods.

The fusion diet embraces the vibrant flavors and culinary traditions of the Mediterranean region, incorporating olive oil, herbs, and spices to enhance the taste of dishes without relying on excessive salt or unhealthy fats. It encourages a balanced and sustainable approach to eating, emphasizing the importance of portion control and mindful eating practices. The fusion of these two renowned dietary patterns provides a comprehensive and effective strategy for individuals seeking to improve their overall health, manage their weight, and reduce their risk of chronic diseases.

Benefits of the Mediterranean DASH Diet

The Mediterranean DASH diet, with its emphasis on fresh produce, lean proteins, and healthy fats, has gained significant attention for its numerous health benefits. This diet, inspired by the traditional eating patterns of Mediterranean countries and the Dietary Approaches to Stop Hypertension (DASH) diet, combines the best of both worlds to create a powerful approach to nutrition. Here's a comprehensive exploration of the benefits of the Mediterranean DASH diet:

1. Improving Heart Health and Lowering Blood Pressure:

One of the primary advantages of the Mediterranean DASH diet is its positive impact on cardiovascular health. By promoting the consumption of heart-healthy foods such as fruits, vegetables, whole grains, and lean proteins, while limiting the intake of saturated fats and refined sugars, this diet aids in reducing the risk of heart disease. Studies have shown that adhering to the Mediterranean DASH diet can help lower blood pressure levels, a significant risk factor for heart-related ailments. The abundance of nutrient-dense foods rich in antioxidants and anti-inflammatory properties helps to protect the heart and improve overall cardiovascular function, leading to a healthier and more resilient cardiovascular system.

2. Managing Weight and Promoting Overall Well-being:

In addition to its cardiovascular benefits, the Mediterranean DASH diet supports weight management and overall well-being. The diet encourages the consumption of whole, unprocessed foods that are naturally low in calories and high in essential nutrients, promoting satiety and reducing the likelihood of overeating. By incorporating a balanced variety of fruits, vegetables, whole grains, and lean proteins, individuals can achieve and maintain a healthy weight, leading to improved energy levels and overall vitality. Furthermore, the diet's focus on wholesome, nutrient-dense foods can contribute to enhanced digestion, better nutrient absorption, and improved overall gut health, fostering a sense of well-being and vitality.

3. Enhancing Cognitive Function and Longevity:

Research has suggested that the Mediterranean DASH diet may play a significant role in promoting cognitive health and longevity. The consumption of foods rich in antioxidants, such as fruits, vegetables, and olive oil, can help combat oxidative stress and inflammation, which are linked to cognitive decline and neurodegenerative diseases. Additionally, the inclusion of omega-3 fatty acids from sources like fish and nuts may support brain health and contribute to improved cognitive function. The diet's focus on maintaining a healthy weight and promoting cardiovascular health also indirectly supports cognitive well-being and may contribute to a longer, healthier life.

In summary, the Mediterranean DASH diet offers a holistic approach to health, providing a wide array of benefits ranging from improved heart health and lowered blood pressure to effective weight management and enhanced cognitive function. By adopting this diet as a lifestyle choice, individuals can embrace a more wholesome and sustainable way of eating, leading to overall well-being and an increased potential for a longer, healthier life.

GETTING STARTED WITH THE MEDITERRANEAN DASH DIET

The Mediterranean DASH Diet combines the principles of the Mediterranean diet and the Dietary Approaches to Stop Hypertension (DASH) diet to create a holistic and healthful approach to eating. By emphasizing nutrient-dense, whole foods and minimizing the intake of processed and high-sodium foods, this diet promotes heart health, weight management, and overall well-being. To embark on your journey with the Mediterranean DASH Diet, it's essential to equip your kitchen with the right pantry staples, ingredients, and tools, and to learn the cooking techniques that will help you create delicious and nourishing meals.

Essential Pantry Staples and Ingredients

1. Extra Virgin Olive Oil: This heart-healthy oil is a cornerstone of the Mediterranean diet, rich in monounsaturated fats and antioxidants.

2. Whole Grains: Stock your pantry with whole grains like quinoa, brown rice, whole wheat pasta, and bulgur for fiber and sustained energy.

3. Legumes: Dried or canned beans, lentils, and chickpeas are excellent sources of plant-based protein, fiber, and essential minerals.

4. Herbs and Spices: Mediterranean herbs such as oregano, basil, thyme, and rosemary, along with spices like cumin, turmeric, and paprika, add robust flavors without the need for excess salt.

5. Nuts and Seeds: Almonds, walnuts, flaxseeds, and chia seeds provide healthy fats, protein, and essential nutrients to your diet.

6. Fresh Produce: Fill your kitchen with a variety of fresh fruits and vegetables, including leafy greens, tomatoes, cucumbers, bell peppers, and citrus fruits.

7. Lean Protein: Incorporate lean sources of protein such as poultry, fish, and plant-based alternatives like tofu and tempeh.

8. Low-fat Dairy: Opt for low-fat or fat-free options of Greek yogurt, cheese, and milk to add calcium and protein to your meals.

9. Canned Tomatoes and Tomato Paste: These can be used in various Mediterranean-inspired dishes like stews, sauces, and soups.

10. Whole Wheat Flour: Use this healthier alternative for baking bread and other baked goods.

Equipment and Cooking Techniques

1. High-Quality Cookware: Invest in quality non-stick pans, pots, and baking sheets for healthier cooking with minimal oil.

2. Blender or Food Processor: These appliances are essential for preparing homemade sauces, dips, and smoothies using fresh and wholesome ingredients.

3. Steamer Basket: Ideal for steaming vegetables while retaining their nutrients and vibrant colors.

4. Grill or Grill Pan: Perfect for grilling fish, poultry, and vegetables, adding a smoky flavor without the need for excess fats.

5. Sharp Knives and Cutting Boards: Ensure you have high-quality knives for chopping, slicing, and dicing various ingredients, and use separate cutting boards for different food groups to prevent cross-contamination.

6. Measuring Tools: Accurate measuring cups and spoons are crucial for portion control and maintaining the balance of ingredients.

7. Oven and Stovetop: Familiarize yourself with different heat settings and cooking methods on your oven and stovetop to prepare a diverse range of Mediterranean-inspired dishes.

8. Mortar and Pestle: Useful for grinding herbs and spices to release their full flavors and aromas.

Cooking Techniques

1. Sautéing: Use minimal oil or broth to cook vegetables and protein for vibrant and flavorful dishes.

2. Baking and Roasting: Enhance the natural flavors of vegetables, fish, and lean meats by baking or roasting them with herbs and spices.

3. Steaming: Preserve the nutrients in vegetables and fish by steaming them until they are tender and flavorful.

4. Grilling: Achieve a charred, smoky taste by grilling vegetables and lean meats to perfection.

5. Homemade Sauces and Dressings: Experiment with homemade sauces and dressings using fresh herbs, olive oil, and citrus juices for a healthier alternative to store-bought options.

6. Meal Prepping: Plan and prepare your meals in advance to ensure you have wholesome and balanced options readily available, making it easier to stick to your Mediterranean DASH Diet plan.

By stocking your kitchen with the necessary pantry items, equipping yourself with the right tools, and mastering these cooking techniques, you'll be well-prepared to create delicious and nourishing Mediterranean-inspired meals that align with the principles of the DASH Diet for a healthier lifestyle.

PART 2:

BREAKFASTS AND BRUNCHES RECIPES

1. *Sweet Potatoes With Coconut Flakes*

Preparation time: 15 mins | Cooking time: 1 hour | Servings: 2

Ingredients:
- 16 ounces of sweet potatoes
- One tablespoon of maple syrup
- ¼ cup of fat-free coconut Greek yogurt
- One eighth cup of toasted coconut flakes, without sugar
- 1 apple, chopped

Direction:
1. Set oven temperature to 400 degrees Fahrenheit.
2. Arrange your potatoes onto a sheet pan. Or until they are tender, bake them for 45 to 60 minutes.
3. Mark the potato "X" with a sharp knife and use a fork to fluff the pulp.
4. Sprinkle maple syrup, Greek yogurt, diced apple, and coconut flakes over top.
5. Serve right away.

Nutrition:
Calories: 321 | Fat: 3 g | Carbs: 70 g | Protein: 7 g | Sugars: 0.1 g | Sodium: 3%

2. *French Toast with Applesauce*

Preparation time: 5 mins | Cooking time: 5 mins | Servings: 6

Ingredients:
- ¼ cup applesauce, unsweetened
- ½ cup skim milk

- 2 teaspoons Stevia
- 2 eggs
- 6 whole wheat bread slices
- 1 teaspoon cinnamon

Directions

1. In a mixing dish, combine applesauce, sugar, cinnamon, milk, and eggs.
2. Soak the bread in the applesauce mixture, one piece at a time, until moist.
3. Heat a large nonstick skillet over medium heat.
4.Place one piece of moistened bread on one side and another on the other. Cook in batches in a single layer for 2-3 minutes per side over medium low heat, or until gently browned.
5. Plate and serve.

**Nutrition information: Calories: 122.6 | Fat: 2.6 g | Carbs: 18.3 g | Protein: 6.5 g
| Sugars: 14.8 g | Sodium: 11%**

3. Baking Powder Biscuits

Preparation time: 5 mins | Cooking time: 5 mins | Servings: 1

Ingredients:
- 1 white egg
- 1 cup white whole wheat flour
- 4 tbsp. Vegetable shortening that is nonhydrogenated
- 1 tablespoon sugar
- 2/3 cup lowfat milk
- 1 cup all-purpose unbleached flour
- 4 tsp. Baking powder with no sodium

Directions

1. Heat the oven to 450°F. Remove a baking sheet from the oven and set it aside.

2. Whisk together the flour, sugar, and baking powder in a large mixing basin.

3. Using your fingertips, cut the shortening into the mixture until it resembles coarse crumbs. Stir in the egg white and milk to mix.

4. Knead the dough for 1 minute on a lightly floured surface. Roll out the dough to a thickness of 3/4 inch and cut it into 12 circles.

5. Arrange the rounds on the baking sheet. Bake for 10 minutes on the center rack of the oven.

6. Remove the baking sheet from the oven and lay the biscuits on a wire rack to cool.

Nutrition: Calories: 118 | Fat:4 g | Carbs:16 g | Protein:3 g | Sugars:0.2 g | Sodium: 6%

4. Oatmeal Banana Pancakes with Walnuts

Preparation time: 15 mins | Cooking time: 5 mins | Servings: 8 pancakes

Ingredients:
- 1 firm banana, coarsely diced
- 1 cup whole wheat pancake batter
- 1/8 cup walnuts, chopped
- 1/4 cup oats, old-fashioned

Directions
1. Prepare the pancake mix according to the package instructions.
2. Stir in the walnuts, oats, and banana chunks.
3. Spray a griddle with nonstick cooking spray. When the griddle is heated, pour approximately 1/4 cup of the pancake batter over it.
4. Flip the pancake when bubbles appear on top. Cook till the top is golden brown.
5. Serve right away.

Nutrition: Calories: 155 | Fat: 4 g | Carbs: 28 g | Protein: 7 g | Sugars: 2.2 g | Sodium: 16%

5. Banana & Cinnamon Oatmeal

Preparation time: 5 mins | Cooking time: 0 mins | Servings: 6

Ingredients:
- 2 cups quick-cook oats
- 4 cups of fat-free milk
- 1 teaspoon cinnamon
- 2 big ripe bananas, chopped
- 4 teaspoons brown sugar
- Cinnamon, extra ground

Directions
1. Heat the milk in a pan over medium heat. Cook for two to four minutes over medium heat, until the oats have thickened. Intermittently stir.
2. Stir in the cinnamon, brown sugar, and banana.
3. If desired, serve with more cinnamon and milk.   Enjoy!

Nutrition Information:
Calories: 215 | Fat:2 g | Carbs:42 g | Protein:10 g | Sugars:1 g | Sodium:40%

6. Avocado Cup with Egg

Preparation time: 5 mins | Cooking time: 0 mins | Servings: 4

Ingredients:
- 4 teaspoons parmesan cheese
- 1 scallion stalk, chopped
- 4 dash pepper
- 4 dash paprika
- 2 avocados, ripe
- 4 large eggs

Directions

1. Preheat the oven to 375 degrees Fahrenheit.
2. Cut avocados in half and remove the seeds.
3. Slice the avocado into spherical pieces to make it level and set comfortably on a baking pan.
4. Place the avocados on a baking sheet and crack one egg into each hole.
5. Evenly season each egg with pepper and paprika.
Bake for 25 minutes, or until the eggs are cooked to your preference.
6. Garnish with parmesan cheese.

Nutrition Information:

Calories: 206 | Fat:15.4 g | Carbs:11.3 g | Protein:8.5 g | Sugars:0.4 g | Sodium:21%

7. Mediterranean Toast

Preparation time: 10 mins | Servings: 2 | Cooking time: 0 mins

Ingredients:

- 1 ½ teaspoon reduced-Fat crumbled feta
- 3 sliced Greek olives
- ¼ mashed avocado
- 1 slice good whole wheat bread
- 1 tablespoon roasted red pepper hummus
- 3 sliced cherry tomatoes
- 1 sliced hard boiled egg

Directions:

1. To begin, toast the bread and spread 1/4 mashed avocado and 1 tablespoon hummus on top.

2. Stir in the cherry tomatoes, olives, hard-boiled egg, and feta cheese.

3. Season with salt and pepper to taste.

Nutrition Information:
Calories: 333.7 | Fat:17 g | Carbs:33.3 g | Protein:16.3 g |Sugars:1 g | Sodium:19%

8. Buckwheat Pancakes with Vanilla Almond Milk

Preparation time: 10 mins | Servings: 1 |Cooking time: 10 mins

Ingredients:
- 1/2 cup vanilla unsweetened almond milk
- 2-4 teaspoons natural sweetener
- 1/8 teaspoon salt
- 1/2 buckwheat flour
- 1/2 teaspoon double-action baking powder

Directions
1. Lightly coat a nonstick pancake griddle with cooking spray and heat over medium heat.
2. In a small mixing bowl, combine the buckwheat flour, salt, baking powder, and stevia, then whisk in the almond milk.
3. Scoop a big spoonful of batter onto the pan and cook until bubbles no longer appear on the surface and the entire surface looks dry (2-4 minutes). Cook for another 2-4 minutes on the other side. Repeat with the rest of the batter.

Nutrition Information
Calories: 240 | Fat:4.5 g | Carbs:2 g | Protein:11 g |Sugars:17 g | Sodium:38%

9. Scrambled Eggs with Mushrooms and Spinach

Preparation time: 5 mins | Servings: 1 | Cooking time: 10 mins

Ingredients:
- 2 beaten egg whites

- 1 whole wheat bread piece
- 1/2 cup fresh sliced mushrooms
- 2 tbsps. Shredded American cheese that is low in fat Pepper
- 1 teaspoon olive oil
- 1 cup fresh spinach, chopped
- 1 complete egg

Directions

1. Heat the oil in a nonstick fry pan over medium high heat. Cover pan with oil and cook for a minute.
2. Stir in the spinach and mushrooms. Cook until the spinach is wilted, about 2-3 minutes.
3. Meanwhile, in a separate dish, mix together the egg whites and cheese. Season with pepper to taste.
4. Pour egg mixture into pan and scramble for 3-4 minutes, or until eggs are cooked through.
5. Serve with a slice of whole wheat bread.

Nutrition Information

Calories: 290.6 | Fat:11.8 g | Carbs:21.8 g | Protein:24.3 g | Sugars:1.4 g | Sodium:24%

10. Mushroom Spinach Omelet

Preparation time: 3 minutes |Cook time: 15 minutes | Servings: 2

Ingredients:
- 1 tbsp. olive oil
- 1/4 cup red onion, sliced
- green onions, diced
- 1 oz. goat cheese
- 1.5 cups fresh spinach
- 5 baby bella mushrooms, sliced
- 1 whole egg; 2 egg whites
- garlic powder, black pepper, to taste.

Directions

1. Heat oil in a medium skillet over medium-high heat.

2. Add red onions and cook for 2-3 minutes. Sauté sliced mushrooms for 4-5 minutes.

3. Add spinach, sauté for about 2 minutes, and season with garlic powder and pepper. Then, leave aside.

4. In a separate dish, whisk together the eggs. Pour the egg mixture into a small pan and cook over medium heat until the eggs are no longer runny.

5. Place the mushroom/spinach mixture on top of the omelet and sprinkle with goat cheese.

6. Fold the omelet in half and cook for 30 seconds more. When the omelet is done, place it on a platter and garnish with green onions.

Nutritional info (per serving):

412 calories | 29.2 g Fat | 18.1 g carbohydrate | 25.2 g Protein | 332 mg Sodium | 25% Fiber.

11. Muesli Scones

Preparation time: 10 minutes | Cook time: 15 minutes | Servings: 16

Ingredients:

- 1 egg
- 1/4 cup dried cranberries
- 1/4 cup chopped dried apricots
- 1/4 cup coarsely chopped pistachios
- 1/4 cup sunflower seeds
- 1/4 cup raw sesame seeds
- 2 tablespoons agave nectar or honey
- 2 cups blanched almond flour (not almond meal)
- 1/2 teaspoon baking soda.

Directions

1. In a mixing dish, combine almond flour and baking soda.

2. Then stir in the dried fruit, seeds, and nuts.

3. In a mixing dish, combine the egg and agave.

4. Mix the egg/agave mixture into the flour/dried fruit mixture with your hands to make a dough.

5. Roll the dough into a 6.5-inch square that is approximately 3/4-inch thick, then cut it into 16 squares.

6. Preheat the oven to 350 degrees Fahrenheit. Bake the dough squares on a baking sheet lined with parchment paper.

Nutritional info (per serving):
76 calories | 5.7 g Fat | 5.0 g carbohydrate | 2.6 gProtein | 106 mg Sodium | 9% Fiber.

12. Sweet Potato Waffles
Preparation time: 5 minutes | Cook time: 10 minutes | Servings: 6

Ingredients:
- 1 banana, sliced
- 1/2 cup sweet potato
- 1 cup oats
- 2 eggs
- 1 cup almond milk
- 1 tablespoon honey
- maple syrup
- 1 tablespoon olive oil
- 1/4 teaspoon baking powder.

Directions

1. In a blender jar, combine all of the ingredients. Blend until completely pureed.

2. Preheat the waffle maker and coat it with cooking spray.

3. Fill each waffle mold with 1/3 cup batter and cook for 3-4 minutes.

4. When finished, drizzle with maple syrup and top with fresh, diced banana.

Nutritional info (per serving):
237 calories | 14.3 g Fat | 24.6 g carbohydrate | 5.1 g Protein | 131 mg Sodium | 3.3 gFiber.

13. Faux Breakfast Hash Brown Cups

Preparation time: 15 mins | Servings: 8 | Cooking time: 0 mins

Ingredients:
- 40 g onion, diced
- 8 medium eggs
- 7½ teaspoon garlic powder
- 2½ g pepper
- 170 g low-fat shredded cheese
- 170 g grated sweet potato
- 2 ½ g salt

Directions
1. Preheat the oven to 400°F and line a muffin pan with paper liners.
2. Mix grated sweet potatoes, onions, garlic, and spices in a basin before spooning one teaspoon into each cup. Place one big egg in each cup and bake for 15 minutes, or until the eggs are done.
3. Serve immediately or save for later.

Nutrition Information:
Calories: 143 | Fat:9.1 g | Carbs:6 g | Protein:9 g Sugars:0 g | Sodium:11%

14. Sweet Corn Muffins
Preparation time: 5 mins | Servings: 1 | Cooking time: 10 mins

Ingredients:
- 1 tablespoon baking powder (sodium-free)
- 3/4 cup non dairy milk
- 1 teaspoon pure vanilla essence

- 1/2 cup sugar
- 1 cup whole-wheat flour
- 1 cup cornmeal
- 1/2 cup canola oil

Directions

1. Preheat the oven to 400 degrees Fahrenheit. Set aside a 12-muffin tray lined with paper liners.
2. Place the cornmeal, flour, sugar, and baking powder into a mixing basin and Whisk well to incorporate.
3. Stir in the non dairy milk, oil, and vanilla extract until mixed.
4. Distribute the batter evenly among the muffin cups. Bake for 15 minutes with the muffin tray on the center rack of the oven.
5. Remove from the oven and cool on a wire rack.

Nutrition Information

Calories: 203 | Fat:9 g | Carbs:26 g | Protein:3 g | Sugars:9.5 g | Sodium:8%

15. Tomato Bruschetta with Basil

Preparation time: 10 mins | Servings: 8 | Cooking time: 10 mins

Ingredients:

- 1/2 cup basil, chopped
- 2 garlic cloves, minced
- 1 tablespoon balsamic vinegar
- 2 tbsps. Extra virgin olive oil
- 12 teaspoon cracked black pepper
- 1 whole wheat baguette, cut
- 8 ripe Roma tomatoes, diced
- 1 teaspoon sea salt

Directions

1. Preheat the oven to 375 degrees Fahrenheit.

2. Dice the tomatoes and combine them with the balsamic vinegar, chopped basil, garlic, salt, pepper, and olive oil in a mixing bowl. Set aside.

3. Slice the baguette into 16-18 pieces and bake for about 10 minutes on a baking sheet.

4. Serve with warm slices of bread and enjoy.

5. Store leftovers in an airtight jar in the refrigerator. Try these over grilled chicken; they're delicious!

Nutrition Information
Calories: 57 | Fat:2.5 g | Carbs:7.9 g | Protein:1.4 g | Sugars:0.2 g | Sodium:12%

LUNCH RECIPES

16. Salad with salmon
Prep Time: 10 minutes | Cooking time: 0 minutes | servings: 3

Ingredients:
- 1 cup flaked canned salmon
- 1 tbsp of lemon juice
- 3 tbsp of yogurt low in fat
- 2 tbsp. chopped red bell pepper
- 1 teaspoon drained and chopped capers
- 1 tablespoon minced red onion
- 1 teaspoon chopped dill
- a pinch of ground black pepper
- 3 slices whole wheat bread

Directions:
1. In a mixing bowl, combine the salmon, lemon juice, yogurt, bell pepper, capers, onion, dill, and black pepper.
2. Spread this on each piece of bread and serve for lunch. Enjoy!

Nutrition information:
calories: 199 |Fat: 2 | Fiber: 4 | Carbs: 14 | 8 g protein | 45% sodium

17. Tuna Salad

Prep Time: 10 minutes | Cooking time: 0 minutes | 3 servings

Ingredients:
- 5 oz. canned tuna in water (drained)
- 1 tablespoon vinegar, red
- 1 tablespoon extra virgin olive oil
- 1/4 cup chopped green onions
- 2 c. arugula

- 1 tbsp. grated low-fat parmesan
- a pinch of ground black pepper
- 2 ounces cooked whole wheat pasta

Directions:
1. Toss the tuna with the vinegar, oil, green onions, arugula, pasta, and black pepper in a mixing bowl.
2. Divide among three dishes, top with parmesan, and serve for lunch. Enjoy!

Nutrition Information:
200 calories | Fat: 4g | Fiber: 4 | Carbs: 14g | 7g protein | 2% sodium

18. Turkey and Mozzarella Sandwich

Prep time: 10 minutes | cooking time: 3 minutes | 2 servings

Ingredients:
2 slices whole wheat bread
2 tsp. mustard
2 smoked turkey slices
1 cored and sliced pear
1/4 cup shredded low-fat mozzarella

Directions:
1. Spread the mustard on each bread slice, split the turkey pieces on one bread slice, add the pear slices and mozzarella, top with the other bread slice, broil for 3 minutes, cut the sandwich in half, and serve. Enjoy!

Nutritional value:
Calories: 171 | Fat: 2g | Fiber: 4g Carbohydrates: 9 | Protein: 9 | Sodium: 16%

19. Veggie Soup

Prep time: 10 minutes | cooking time: 16 minutes | 6 servings

Ingredients:
- 2 tbsp. olive oil
- 1½ cup shredded carrot
- 6 minced garlic cloves
- 1 cup chopped yellow onion
- 1 cup chopped celery
- 32 ounces low-sodium chicken stock
- 4 c. water
- 1½ cup whole wheat pasta
- 1/4 cup low-fat parmesan, grated
- 2 tablespoons parsley, chopped

Directions
1. Heat the oil in a saucepan over medium-high heat, then add the garlic, stir, and cook for 1 minute.
2. Cook for 7 minutes after adding the onion, carrot, and celery.
3. Stir in the stock, water, and pasta, then bring to a boil over medium heat for 8 minutes.
4. Serve in dishes, garnished with parsley and parmesan. Enjoy!

Nutritional information
Calories: 212 | Fat: 4 | Fiber: 4 | Carbohydrates: 13 | Protein: 8 | Sodium: 17%

20. Spaghetti Squash with Sauce

Time to prepare: 10 minutes | Time to cook: 25 minutes | 4 servings

Ingredients:
- 1 pound of ground beef

- 1/2 cup yellow onion, chopped
- 1/2 cup green bell pepper, chopped
- 2 garlic cloves, minced
- 14 ounces canned no-salt-added tomatoes, chopped
- 2 tbsp tomato paste
- 8 oz. tomato sauce
- 1 teaspoon of Italian seasoning
- 1/4 cup shredded low-fat parmesan
- 2 pounds spaghetti squash, pierced with a knife

Directions:

1. Place the spaghetti squash on a prepared baking sheet and bake at 400 degrees F for 10 minutes. Cut into halves, shred and divide the squash pulp into spaghetti, and place in a bowl.

2. Heat a skillet over medium-high heat, then add the meat and brown for 5 minutes, stirring occasionally.

3. Cook for 10 minutes after adding the onion, bell pepper, garlic, tomatoes, tomato paste, tomato sauce, and Italian seasoning.

4. Divide the squash spaghetti among dishes, top with the meat mixture, and serve with parmesan. Enjoy!

Nutritional information
Calories: 231 | Fat: 4 | Fiber: 5 | Carbohydrates: 14 | Protein: 9 | Sodium: 24%

21. Salad with Shrimp

Time to prepare: 10 minutes | Time to cook: 8 minutes | 4 servings

Ingredients:
- 12 ounces trimmed and halved asparagus spears
- 8 oz. infant corn
- 12 endive leaves,
- 12 baby lettuce leaves, ripped

- 12 spinach leaves
- 12 ounces cooked, peeled, and deveined shrimp
- 2½ cup red raspberries
- ¼ cup raspberry vinegar
- ¼ cup olive oil
- 1 tablespoon chopped cilantro
- 2 teaspoons stevia

Directions:

1. Fill a saucepan halfway with water, bring to a boil over medium-high heat, add asparagus, simmer for 8 minutes, transfer to a dish of cold water, cool, drain thoroughly, and place in a salad bowl. Corn, endive leaves, spinach, lettuce, prawns, and raspberries may all be added.

2. In a separate bowl, mix together the oil, vinegar, stevia, and cilantro. Add to your salad, stir, and serve for lunch. Enjoy!

Nutritional Information
Calories: 199 | Fat: 2 | Fiber: 3 | Carbohydrates: 14 | Protein: 8 | Sodium: 54%

22. Tacos de Pollo (chicken tacos)

Time to prepare: 10 minutes | Time to cook: 0 minutes | 2 servings

Ingredients:
- 4 mini taco shells
- 2 tablespoons chopped celery
- 1 tbsp. light mayonnaise
- 1 teaspoon salsa
- 1 tablespoon shredded low-fat cheddar
- 1/3 cup cooked and shredded chicken

Directions:

1. Toss the celery with the mayo, salsa, cheddar, and chicken in a mixing dish.
2. Fill tiny taco shells with this mixture and serve for lunch. Enjoy!

Nutritional value:
Calories: 221 | Fat: 3 | Fiber: 8 | Carbohydrates: 14 | Protein: 9 | Sodium: 48%

23. *Lunch Salad with Quinoa and Spinach*

Time to prepare: 10 minutes | Time to cook: 25 minutes | 4 servings

Ingredients:
- 1 cup quinoa
- 2 tsp. olive oil
- 1/2 cup dried and chopped apricots
- 2 minced garlic cloves
- 2 cups water
- A pinch of ground black pepper
- 1 cup halved cherry tomatoes
- 1 chopped red onion
- 8 cups fresh baby spinach
- 1/4 cup sliced almonds

To make the salad dressing:
1/2 teaspoon grated lemon zest
2 tbsp of lemon juice
1 tsp. coconut sugar
1/2 tsp Dijon mustard
four tbsp olive oil

Directions
1. Heat a skillet over medium heat, add the quinoa, toast for 5 minutes, and transfer to a bowl.

2. Heat the oil in a pan over medium heat, then add the garlic and cook for 1 minute, stirring constantly.
3. Cook for 4 minutes longer after adding the quinoa and apricots.
4. Bring to a boil, then reduce to a simmer for another 15 minutes.
5. Combine the tomatoes, onion, spinach, almonds, quinoa, and apricots in a salad dish.
6. In a separate dish, mix together the lemon zest, lemon juice, sugar, mustard, and oil. Add to the quinoa salad, stir, and serve for lunch. Enjoy!

Nuttritional information
Calories: 199, Fat: 3, Fiber: 4, Carbohydrates: 16, Protein: 8, Sodium: 4%

24. Chinese Chicken
Time to prepare: 10 minutes | time to cook: 10 minutes | 4 servings

Ingredients:
- 5 lbs chicken thighs
- ½ cup balsamic vinegar
- 1 teaspoon black peppercorns, dried
- 1/2 cup of coconut aminos
- black pepper for flavor
- 4 minced garlic cloves.

Directions:
1. In the instant pot, combine the chicken, vinegar, aminos, garlic, pepper, and peppercorns. Combine everything.
2. Then, heat it for 15 minutes on high.
3. Divide it up and serve!

Nutritional Information:
261 calories | Carbohydrates: 18g | Net Carbohydrates: 10g | Fiber: 8g | Protein: 8g | Sodium: 33%.

25. Insrant pot Beef Gyros

Time to prepare: 10 minutes | time to cook: 15 minutes | 6 servings

Ingredients:
- 2 pounds thinly sliced beef roast
- 1 tbsp. dry parsley
- 1 teaspoon sea salt
- 3 minced garlic cloves
- 1 teaspoon ground black pepper
- 1 red onion, sliced
- 4 tablespoons preferred oil
- 1 tablespoon of olive oil
- 1/2 cup vegetable broth
- 1 tsp lemon juice

To make the Tzatziki sauce:
- 1 cup unsweetened yogurt
- 1 minced garlic clove
- 2 teaspoons fresh dill
- 12 cup cucumber, peeled, seeded, and coarsely chopped

Directions:
1. Turn on the instant pot and pour the oil to the bottom.
2. To sear and soften the onions, add the meat, spices, garlic, and onion.
3. Pour the lemon juice and broth over the meat, mix it, lock the cover in place, and then use meat/stew for 9 minutes.
4. Allow it to naturally release pressure for 3 minutes before releasing it quickly.
5. If you wish to add veggie toppings or apple cider vinegar to the Tzatziki sauce, do so.
6. Before adding meat and garnishes, place lettuce in the bottom of naan or pita bread.

Nutrition Information:
395 calories | Fat: 27g | Carbohydrates: 4g | 4g net carbs
| 32g protein | 0g fiber. | 38% sodium

26. Pasta with Meat Sauce

Time to prepare: 10 minutes | time to | cook: 5 minutes | 4-6 servings

Ingredients:
- 2 minced garlic cloves
- 1 red pepper, chopped
- 8 ounces dried pasta
- 1/2 ounces of water
- 1 small onion, chopped
- 2 lbs ground meat
- 1 jar spaghetti sauce

Directions:
1. Set the instant pot to sauté mode.
2. Cook until the onions, peppers, and meat are no longer pink.
3. Stir in the pasta, spaghetti sauce, and water.
4. Set it to manual for 5 minutes, then fast release, and top with cheese and parsley.

Nutrition Information:
437 calories | Fat: 25g. | Carbohydrates: 30g | Net Carbohydrates: 26g | 24g protein | 4g fiber | 6% sodium

27. Instant pot Egg Sandwiches

**Time to prepare: 5 minutes; time to cook: 10 minutes
2 servings**

Ingredients:

- 2 baguettes, brown
- 6 tablespoons of mayonnaise
- 1/2 cup fresh onion
- 1 teaspoon ground mustard powder
- To taste, add butter, salt, and pepper.
- six huge eggs
- 1/2 cup cucumbers
- 1 big carrot
- 1/2 cup shredded cheese
- 1 teaspoon fresh parsley

Directions:

1. Put a cup of water in the bottom, then steam the eggs for 5 minutes in steamer baskets.

2. Prepare your carrot, dice your cucumber and onion, grate cheese, and combine all ingredients except the spring onion in a mixing bowl, seasoning and adding mayonnaise to combine. After cutting the baguettes in half, take the eggs and place them in cold water, shells removed.

3. Mash the eggs with the other ingredients to make an egg mayonnaise, and then brown the bread with butter as desired.

4. Sauté the spring onion, then stack the toast, mayonnaise mixture, and spring onions, and serve!

Nutritional Information:
260 calories Fat: 13g | Carbohydrates: 38g | 31g net carbs | 33g protein | 7g fiber | 19% sodium

28. Teriyaki Chicken

Time to prepare: 8 minutes | time to cook: 22 minutes | 4 servings

Teriyaki sauce ingredients:
- 1/3 cup soy sauce (low salt)
- 1/4 cup of honey

- 1/4 cup rice wine vinegar or apple cider vinegar 3 tbsp arrowroot powder or corn starch
- 1/4 teaspoon sherry or mirin
- 3 tbsp water for the sauce

For chicken with rice:
- 1 tablespoon olive oil or toasted sesame oil
- season with salt and black pepper to taste
- 1/2 teaspoon ginger, chopped or grated
- 1/3 cup carrots, shredded
- 1 cup of water
- 1/3 cup shelled edamame beans, defrosted, chopped green onions
- 1 boneless, skinless medium chicken breast
- 2 minced garlic cloves
- 14 cup diced red bell peppers
- 2 cups cleaned, rinsed, and drained uncooked Jasmine rice
- 1 cup florets broccoli
- Topping: sesame seeds

Directions:
1. Then, heat the oil and add the chicken, seasoned with salt and pepper and sautéing for 2-3 minutes, until browned.
2. Cook for 20 seconds after adding the ginger and garlic.
3. Pour half of the sauce and one cup of water into uncooked rice.
4. Cook on high pressure for 3 minutes, then release the pressure naturally.
5. Add the vegetables and whisk up the cornstarch slurry, then spread it over the chicken and simmer until the vegetables are soft, then sprinkle with seeds and green onions and serve hot.

Nutritional information:
419 calories | Fat: 6g Carbohydrates: 81g | 79g net carbs | 8g protein | 2g Fiber | 64% Sodium

29. Pasta with Tuscan Chicken

Time to prepare: 10 minutes | time to cook: 4 minutes | 6 servings

Ingredients:

- 1/2 tbsp Italian spice
- 3 cups low-sodium chicken broth
- 12 oz. Noodles made with whole wheat
- 1 c. cottage cheese
- 1/4 teaspoon black pepper
- ⅓ Sun-dried tomatoes
- 1 tbsp. minced garlic
- 2 lbs chicken breast
- 2 c. spinach
- 1 cup Greek yogurt, plain
- 1/4 cup Parmesan and 1/4 cup basil

Directions:

1. Turn the IP to sauté and toss in the tomatoes, garlic, seasoning pepper, and salt for 30 seconds.
2. Brown the chicken for 1-2 minutes, stirring often to prevent it from sticking.
3. Stir in the noodles and chicken broth to coat.
4. Cook for 4 minutes on manual, then quickly remove the pressure, but be cautious.
5. Set aside the yogurt and cottage cheese mixture.
6. Stir the spaghetti and noodles together, then add the cheese, basil, and spinach and mix well.
7. Pour cream over spaghetti and toss until evenly coated.

Nutritional Information:

479 calories | Fat: 9g | Carbohydrates: 49g | Net Carbohydrates: 48g | 54g protein | 1g fiber | 52% sodium

Time to prepare: 5 minutes | time to cook: 30 minutes | 4 servings

Ingredients:
- 1 cup dry black beans (no need to soak)
- 1 chipotle pepper from an adobo sauce can
- 1/2 tsp dried oregano
- Sea salt
- 3 c. water
- 1 tsp cumin
- 1 c. brown rice
- **Toppings:** lime and cilantro

Directions:
1. Add the beans, water, pepper, cumin, and oregano, and then add the rice, salt, and approximately 1¼ cups of water to an oven-safe bowl, and place the trivet and rice on top.
2. From here, secure the lead, seal it, and hand cook it for 3-0 minutes. Once completed, vent it and let it naturally release pressure.
3. Remove everything, and then mash the beans together with a masher and season them to taste.
4. Serve with your preferred burrito bowl toppings.

Nutritional information:
339 calories | Fat: 2g
 | Carbohydrates: 66g | 54g net carbs | 15g protein | 9g fiber | 1% sodium .

DINNER

31. Goat Cheese Fold-Overs

Time to prepare: 15 minutes | Time to cook: 8 minutes | 4 servings

Ingredients:
- 8 oz crumbled goat cheese
- 5 oz sliced ham
- 1/4 cup coconut milk
- 1 cup almond flour
- 1 tsp. of olive oil
- 1 teaspoon Italian seasoning
- 1/2 teaspoon dried dill
- 1/2 teaspoon of salt

Directions:
1. Combine almond flour, coconut milk, olive oil, and salt in a mixing bowl. The batter will be silky.
2. Preheat a nonstick skillet over medium heat.
3. Divide the batter into four equal portions. Pour the first batter portion onto the hot pan and cook for 1 minute on each side.
4. Repeat with the remaining batter.
5. After that, combine crumbled goat cheese, dried dill, and Italian spice in a mixing bowl.
6. Spread the goat cheese mixture over each almond flour pancake. 7. Fold in the slices of ham.

Nutritional Information
caloric intake: 402 | Sodium 69% | Fat 31.8 | Fiber 1.6 | Carbohydrates 5.1 | Protein 25.1

**Time to prepare: 15 minutes
| Time to cook: 25 minutes | 4 servings**

Ingredients:
- 1 quart coconut milk
- 2 quarts of water
- 1 tsp curry paste
- 4 thighs of chicken
- 1/2 teaspoon grated fresh ginger
- 1 minced garlic clove
- 1 tsp. butter
- 1 tsp chili flakes
- 1 tablespoon of lemon juice

Directions:
1. Melt the butter in a pan over medium heat.
2. Add the garlic and ginger, diced. Cook for 1 minute with the ingredients. They must be continually stirred.
3. Fill the pot halfway with water. Pour in the coconut milk and curry paste. Mix the liquid until it is homogeneous.
4. Combine the chicken thighs, chili flakes, and cooked ginger mixture in a mixing bowl. Cook the soup for 15 minutes with the lid closed.
5. Then, using a hand whisker, begin whisking the soup and adding the lemon juice.
6. Stop whisking after all of the lemon juice has been added. Cook the soup for 5 minutes longer over medium heat with the lid closed.
7. Then take the soup from the heat and let it aside for 15 minutes to cool.

Nutritional information:
318 calories | 26g fat | 1.4g fiber | 4.2 carbs | 20.6g protein | 14% sodium

Time to prepare: 10 minutes | Time to cook: 5 minutes | 4 servings

Ingredients:
- 4 lettuce leaves
- 1/2 diced red onion
- 1/2 minced jalapeño pepper
- 1 tablespoon extra virgin olive oil
- 1 pound fillet cod
- 1 tablespoon of lemon juice
- 1/4 teaspoon coriander powder

Directions:
1. 1/2 tbsp olive oil and powdered coriander should be sprinkled over the fish filet.
2. Preheat the grill to high heat.
3. Grill for 2 minutes on each side of the fish. The hue of the cooked fish is light brown.
4. Following that, combine the diced red onion, minced jalapeño pepper, remaining olive oil, and lemon juice.
5. Divide the grilled fish filet into four pieces.
6. Wrap the fish in lettuce leaves. Place the tacos on serving plates and top with the combined red onion mixture.

Nutritional Information
Calories: 157 | Fat: 4.5 | Fiber: 0.4 | Carbs: 1.6 | Protein: 26.1 | Sodium: 37%

34. Cobb Salad

Time to prepare: 10 minutes
| Time to cook: 5 minutes
| 2 servings

Ingredients:
- 2 oz. sliced bacon
- 1 cooked egg, peeled
- 1/2 tomato, chopped
- 1 pound blue cheese
- 1 teaspoon chopped chives
- 1/3 cup chopped lettuce
- 1 tablespoon of mayonnaise
- 1 tablespoon of lemon juice

Directions:
1. Place the bacon in the hot skillet and cook for 1.5 minutes on each side.
2. When the bacon is done, coarsely cut it and place it in the salad dish.
Add the chopped eggs to the salad dish as well.
3. Then, add the chopped tomato, chives, and lettuce.
4. Chop the Blue cheese and toss it into the salad.
5. Then, prepare the seasoning by whisking together mayonnaise and lemon juice.
6. Pour the dressing over the salad and gently shake.

Nutritional information
270 calories| 20.7g fat | 0.3g fiber | 3.7 carbs | 16.6g protein | 43% sodium

35. Clam Chowder

Time to prepare: 5 minutes | Time to cook: 15 minutes | 3 servings

Ingredients:
- 1 quart coconut milk
- 1 quart of water
- 6 ounces. chopped clam
- 1 teaspoon chopped chives

- 1/2 tsp white pepper
- a quarter teaspoon chili flakes
- 1/2 teaspoon of salt
- 1 cup chopped broccoli florets

Directions:

1. In a saucepan, combine the coconut milk and water.

2. Combine the clams, chives, white pepper, chili flakes, salt, and broccoli florets in a mixing bowl.

3. Close the lid and boil the chowder for 15 minutes, or until all of the ingredients are tender.

4. It is best to serve the soup hot.

Nutritional information

Calories 139 | Fat 9.8 | Fiber 1.1 | Carbohydrates 10.8 | Protein 2.4 | Sodium 44%

36. Carbonara

Time to prepare: 10 minutes | Time to cook: 25 minutes | 6 servings

Ingredients:
- 3 trimmed zucchini
- 1 quart thick cream
- 5 ounces chopped bacon
- 2 egg yolks
- 4 oz. grated Cheddar cheese
- 1 tablespoon melted butter
- 1 tsp. chili flakes
- 1 teaspoon sea salt
- 1/2 cup cooking water

Directions:

1. Spiralize the zucchini to make zucchini noodles.

2. Toss the bacon in the pan and cook for 5 minutes on medium heat. 3. From time to time, give it a good stir.

4. Meanwhile, combine heavy cream, butter, salt, and chili flakes in a saucepan.

5. Whisk in the egg yolk until the mixture is smooth.

6. Begin heating the liquid, stirring regularly.

7. When the liquid begins to boil, stir in the grated cheese and cooked bacon. Close the cover and mix everything together. Cook for 5 minutes over low heat.

8. Meanwhile, bake the zucchini noodles in the pan where the bacon was for 3 minutes.

9. Then, pour the heavy cream mixture over the zucchini and combine. Cook for 1 minute longer before transferring to serving plates.

Nutritional information:
calories 324 | Fat 27.1 | Fiber 1.1 | Carbs 4.6 | Protein 16 | Sodium 65%

37. Seeded Cauliflower Soup
Time to prepare: 10 minutes | Time to cook: 20 minutes | 4 servings

Ingredients:
- 2 cups cauliflower
- 1 tbsp. pumpkin seeds
- 1 tbsp chia seeds
- 1/2 tsp. of salt
- 1 tsp. butter
- 1/4 diced white onion
- 1/2 cup coconut cream
- 1 quart of water
- 4 ounces grated Parmesan
- 1 tsp. paprika
- 1 tbsp. dried cilantro

Directions:
1. Chop the cauliflower and put it in a pot.
2. Season with salt, butter, onion, paprika, and dried cilantro.
3. Cook the cauliflower for 5 minutes on medium heat.
4. Then stir in the coconut cream and water.
5. Close the top and bring the soup to a boil for 15 minutes.
6. The soup should then be blended using a hand blender.
7. Dring to re-boil it.
8. Mix in the grated cheese well.
9. Pour the soup into serving cups and sprinkle with pumpkin seeds and chia seeds.

Nutritional information
214 calories | 16.4g fat | 3.6g fiber | 8.1g carbohydrates| 12.1g protein | 43% sodium

38. Asparagus Wrapped in Prosciutto
Time to prepare: 15 minutes | Time to cook: 20 minutes | 6 servings

Ingredients:
- 2 pounds of asparagus
- 8 ounces. sliced prosciutto
- 1/2 teaspoon powdered black pepper
- 1 tablespoon melted butter
- 4 tablespoons thick cream
- 1 tablespoon of lemon juice

Directions:
1. Prosciutto slices should be cut into strips.
2. Arrange asparagus on a tray wrapped in prosciutto slices.
3. Season the veggies with black pepper, heavy cream, and lemon juice to taste. Add the butter.
4. Preheat the oven to 365 degrees Fahrenheit.
5. Place the asparagus tray in the oven and bake for 20 minutes.

6. Only serve the prepared food hot.

Nutritional information
**Calories 138 | Fat 7.9 | Fiber 3.2 | Carbs 6.9 | Protein 11.5 |
Sodium 3%**

39. Stuffed Bell Peppers

**Time to prepare: 10 minutes | Time to cook: 25 minutes
| 4 servings**

Ingredients:
- 4 bell peppers
- 1½ pound ground beef
- 1 grated zucchini
- 1 diced white onion
- 1/2 tsp ground nutmeg
- 1 tablespoon extra virgin olive oil
- 1 teaspoon black pepper, ground
- 1/2 teaspoon of salt
- 3 oz. grated Parmesan 1.

Directions:
1. Remove the seeds from the bell peppers and cut them in half.
2. In a skillet, brown the ground meat.
3. Combine the grated zucchini, diced onion, ground nutmeg, olive oil, ground black pepper, and salt in a mixing bowl.
4. For 5 minutes, roast the mixture.
Fill the tray with bell pepper halves.
5. Fill each pepper half halfway with the ground beef mixture and sprinkle with grated Parmesan.
6. Wrap the tray with foil and tape the edges shut.
7. Cook the filled bell peppers for 20 minutes at 360 degrees Fahrenheit.

Nutritional information
Calories: 241 | Fat: 14.6 | Fiber: 3.4 | Carbs: 11| Protein: 18.6 | 37% sodium

40. Zucchini Bars

Time to prepare: 10 minutes | Time to cook: 15 minutes | 8 servings

Ingredients:
- ½ diced white onion
- 3 grated zucchini
- 2 tsp. butter
- 3 whisked eggs
- 4 tbsp coconut flour
- 1 teaspoon sea salt
- 1/2 teaspoon black pepper, ground
- 5 oz crumbled goat cheese
- 1/2 cup chopped spinach
- 4 ounce crumbled Swiss cheese
- 1 tsp. baking powder
- 1/2 tsp lemon juice

Directions:
1. Combine grated zucchini, diced onion, eggs, coconut flour, salt, powdered black pepper, crumbled cheese, chopped spinach, baking powder, and lemon juice in a mixing dish.
2. Stir in the butter until the mixture is homogeneous.
3. Line a baking dish with parchment paper.
4. Place the zucchini mixture in the baking dish and press it down.
5. Preheat the oven to 365 degrees Fahrenheit and place the dish inside.
6. Cooking time is 15 minutes. The food should then be thoroughly chilled.
7. Make it into bars.

Nutritional information:

199 calories | 1316 fat | 215 fiber | 7.1 carbs |13.1 protein | 21% sodium

41. Merjimek
**Time to prepare: 7 minutes | Time to cook: 40 minutes
| 4 servings**

Ingredients:
- 1 pound red lentils
- 1 teaspoon pepper paste 3 tablespoons sunflower oil
- 1/2 tsp chili pepper
- 1/2 teaspoon chili flakes
- 1/2 teaspoon of salt
- 1 tbsp. butter
- 1/2 tsp. paprika
- 1/2 teaspoon black pepper, ground
- 4 c. of water
- 1 chopped green pepper
- 2 finely chopped potatoes

Directions:
1. Melt the butter in a saucepan.
2. Roast the vegetables for 5 minutes over medium heat with chopped pepper and potatoes. They should be stirred every now and again.
3. Add water, lentils, ground black pepper, paprika, salt, chili flakes, chili pepper, pepper paste, and oil after that. Using the spoon, combine the ingredients.
4. Cook the soup for 35 minutes on medium heat with the lid closed.
5. The prepared soup should have the texture of a soft purée.

Nutritional information
Calories 354 | Fat 12.2 | Fiber 18 | Carbohydrates 47.7 | Protein 14.6

42. Chicken Leek soup

**Time to prepare: 10 minutes | Time to cook: 35 minutes
| 4 servings**

Ingredients:
- 1 cup shredded cabbage
- 6 ounces chopped leek
- 1/2 diced yellow onion
- 1 pound skinless, boneless chicken breast
- 1 tablespoon melted butter
- 1 teaspoon sea salt
- 1/2 tsp dried oregano
- 1/2 tsp dried thyme
- 1 teaspoon of canola oil
- 4 cups of water

Directions:
1. Place the chicken breast in the pan, cut into pieces.
2. Combine the butter and canola oil.
Cook for 5 minutes the chicken. From time to time, give it a good stir.
After that, add the chopped leek and yellow onion.
3. Season with salt, dried oregano, and thyme. Combine the ingredients and sauté for 5 minutes.
4. Then add the cabbage and water.
Close the cover and simmer the soup for 25 minutes on medium heat.

Nutritional information
Calories 222 | Fat 9.4 | Fiber 1.6 | Carbs 8.5| Protein 25.1

Time to prepare: 10 minutes | Time to cook: 30 minutes | 4 servings

Ingredients:
- 1 pound ground beef
- 1 tbsp. semolina
- 1/2 teaspoon of salt
- 1 yolk of an egg
- 1/2 teaspoon black pepper, ground
- 4 cup chicken broth
- 1 sliced carrot
- 1 diced yellow onion
- 1 tablespoon melted butter
- 1/2 tablespoon turmeric
- 1/2 tsp garlic powder

Directions:
1. Heat the butter in the pan until it has melted. Cook until the onion is light brown. Meanwhile, add the chicken stock to the pan. Mix in the garlic powder and turmeric.
2. Bring the water to a boil. Boil for 10 minutes with diced carrot.
3. Combine ground beef, semolina, salt, egg yolk, and ground black pepper in a mixing bowl.
4. Make the meatballs in tiny sizes.
Place the meatballs in a bowl with the chicken stock.
5. Cooked onion should be added now.
6. Cook the soup over medium-low heat for 15 minutes.

Nutritional information
Calories: 143 | Fat: 8.8 | Fiber: 1.2 | Carbs: 7.5 | Protein: 8.8

Time to prepare: 10 minutes | Time to cook: 50 minutes | 8 servings

Ingredients:
- 1½ pound lamb bone
- 4 beaten eggs
- 2 cups chopped lettuce
- 1/2 cup fresh dill, diced
- 1 tablespoon chopped chives,
- 1/2 cup lemon juice
- 1 teaspoon sea salt
- 1/2 tsp white pepper
- 2 teaspoons avocado oil
- 5 quarts of water

Directions:
1. Place the lamb in the pan, coarsely chopped.
2. Roast the meat for 10 minutes over medium heat with avocado oil.
3. From time to time, stir it with a spatula.
4. Then season the meat with salt and white pepper. Bring the mixture to a boil by adding water.
5. Whisk together the eggs and lemon juice in a mixing basin.
6. Whisk in 12 cup of the pan's hot water until the egg mixture is smooth.
In the soup, combine dill, chives, and lettuce. Stir well.
7. Cook the soup over medium-high heat for 30 minutes.
8. Then add the egg mixture and quickly toss it in to ensure that the soup has a uniform texture.
9. Cook for another 3 minutes.

Nutritional information:
Calories: 360 | Fat: 22.9 | Fiber: 0.8 | Carbohydrates: 2.9 | Protein: 33.6

45. Eggplant soup

Time to prepare: 10 minutes | Time to cook: 30 minutes | 4 servings

Ingredients:
- 1/2 cup chopped tomatoes
- 2 trimmed eggplants
- 1/4 cup fresh parsley, chopped
- 1/4 cup fresh cilantro, diced
- 1 yellow onion
- 1/2 teaspoon cumin powder
- 1/2 tsp cayenne pepper
- 1 sliced celery stalk
- 1 tablespoon extra virgin olive oil
- 1 teaspoon sea salt
- 1 peeled garlic clove
- 1 tbsp. butter
- 4 cup chicken broth

Directions:
1. Peel the eggplants and season with salt and olive oil.
2. Preheat the oven to 360 degrees Fahrenheit.
3. Place the eggplants on the baking pan and place it in the preheated oven.
4. Cook the veggies for 25 minutes in the oven.
5. Meanwhile, add the chicken stock to the pan.
6. Chop the tomatoes, parsley, cilantro, cumin, cayenne pepper, celery stem, and garlic clove.
7. Allow the mixture to simmer for 5 minutes.
8. Meanwhile, melt the butter in a pan over medium heat.
9. Roast the onion until it is transparent.
10. Combine the boiling chicken stock with the onion.
11. When the eggplants are done, place them in a food processor and puree until smooth.

12. Following that, add the pureed eggplants to the chicken stock combination.

13. Blend the soup with a hand blender until it has a creamy texture.

14. Cook the soup for 5 minutes on low heat.

Nutritional information:
137 calories | 5.7 grams of fat | 10.9 grams of fiber | 21.2 grams of carbs | 4.2 grams of protein

46. Meatballs platters

4 servings |Time to prepare: 10 minutes| Time to cook: 15 minutes

Ingredients:
- 1 pound ground beef
- 1/4 cup panko breadcrumbs
- a sprinkle of black pepper and salt
- 1/4 cup parsley, chopped
- 3 tablespoons red onion, shredded
- 2 garlic cloves, minced
- 2 tbsp of lemon juice
- 1 lemon zest
- 1 egg, grated
- 1/2 teaspoon cumin,
- 1/2 teaspoon coriander
- 1/4 teaspoon cinnamon powder
- 2 oz. crumbled feta cheese

Directions:
1. In a mixing bowl, combine the meat, breadcrumbs, salt, pepper, and the other ingredients (excluding the cooking spray), toss well, and form into medium balls.
2. Place the meatballs on a baking sheet lined with parchment paper, coat with cooking spray, and bake for 15 minutes at 450°F.
3. Serve the meatballs as an appetizer on a dish.

Nutritional information:
300 calories | 15.4 g fat | 6.4 g fiber | 22.4 g carbs | 35 g protein

47. Bruschetta with Tomatoes

6 servings | Time to prepare: 10 minutes | Time to cook: 10 minutes

Ingredients:
- 1 sliced baguette,
- 1/3 cup chopped basil
- 6 cubed tomatoes
- 2 garlic minced cloves
- a sprinkle of black pepper and salt
- 1 teaspoon of olive oil
- 1 tbsp. balsamic vinegar
- 1/2 tsp garlic powder
- Spray cooking oil

Directions:
1. Place the baguette slices on a baking sheet lined with parchment paper, coat with cooking spray, and bake for 10 minutes at 400° F.
2. Toss the tomatoes with the basil and the other ingredients in a mixing basin for 10 minutes.
3. Divide the tomato mixture among the baguette slices, put on a tray, and serve.

Nutritional information: 162 calories | 4 g fat | 7 g fiber | 29 g carbohydrates | 4 g protein

48. Red Pepper Tapenade

4 servings | Time to prepare: 10 minutes | Time to cook: 0 minutes

Ingredients:
- 7 ounces chopped roasted red peppers
- 1/2 cup grated parmesan
- 1/3 cup chopped parsley

- 14 ounces canned artichokes, drained and diced
- 3 tablespoons olive oil
- 1/4 cup drained capers
- 11½ tablespoon lemon juice
- 2 minced garlic cloves

Direction:

1. In a blender, add the red peppers, parmesan, and other ingredients and pulse until smooth.
2. Serve as a snack in individual cups.

Nutritional information:

200 calories | 5.6 g fat | 4.5 g fiber | 12.4 g carbs | 4.6 g protein

49. Salsa de Chili Mango y Watermelon

12 servings | Time to prepare: 5 minutes | Time to cook: 0 minutes

Ingredients:

- 1 chopped red tomato
- To taste, season with salt and black pepper.
- 1 cup seedless watermelon, peeled and cubed
- 1 sliced red onion
- 2 peeled and cut mangos
- 1/4 cup chopped cilantro
- 2 chile chopped peppers
- 3 tablespoons lime juice
- Pita chips to serve

Directions:

1. Toss the tomato, watermelon, onion, and other ingredients (except the pita chips) in a mixing dish. Serve the mixture in tiny cups with pita chips on the side.

Nutritional information:
62 calories | 1.3 g fiber | 3.9 g carbohydrates | 2.3 g protein

50. Hummus with Red Peppers
6 servings | Time to prepare: 10 minutes | Time to cook: 0 minutes

Ingredients:
- 6 ounces peeled and diced roasted red peppers
- 16 ounces washed and drained canned chickpeas
- 1/4 cup plain Greek yogurt
- 3 tbsp tahini paste
- 1 lemon juice
- 3 minced garlic cloves
- 1 tablespoon extra virgin olive oil
- a sprinkle of black pepper and salt
- 1 tablespoon chopped parsley

Directions:
1. In a food processor, mix the red peppers with the other ingredients (excluding the oil and parsley) and pulse until thoroughly combined.
2. Add the oil, pulse one more, divide into cups, garnish with parsley, and serve as a party spread.

Nutritional information:
Calories: 255 | Fat: 11.4 g | Fiber: 4.5 g | Carbohydrates: 17.4 g | Protein: 6.5 g

51. Eggplant Dip
4 servings |Time to prepare: 10 minutes | Time to cook: 40 minutes

Ingredients:
- 1 eggplant, prickly with a fork
- 2 tbsp of tahini paste

- 2 tbsp of lemon juice
- 2 minced garlic cloves
- 1 tablespoon extra virgin olive oil
- To taste, season with salt and black pepper.
- 1 tablespoon chopped parsley

Directions:

1. Place the eggplant in a roasting pan and bake at 400° F for 40 minutes. Allow to cool before peeling and transferring to a food processor.

2. Add the other ingredients, except the parsley, and blend until smooth. 3. Divide into small bowls and serve as an appetizer, garnished with the parsley.

Nutritional information:

121 calories | 4.3 g fat | 1 g fiber | 1.4 g carbs | 4.3 g protein

52. Cucumber Bites

12 servings | Time to prepare: 10 minutes | Time to cook: 0 minutes

Ingredients

- 1 English cucumber, thinly cut into 32 rounds
- 10 oz. hummus
- 16 halved cherry tomatoes
- 1 tablespoon minced parsley
- 1 ounce crumbled feta cheese

Directions:

1. Spread the hummus on each cucumber round, then split the tomato halves on top, sprinkle with cheese and parsley, and serve as an appetizer.

Nutritional information: 162 calories | 3.4 g fat | 2 g fiber | 6.4 g carbs | 2.4 g protein

53. Cucumber Rolls
6 servings | Time to prepare: 5 minutes | Time to cook: 0 minutes

Ingredients:
- 1 large cucumber, cut in half lengthwise
- 1 tablespoon chopped parsley
- 8 ounces canned tuna, drained and mashed
- To taste, season with salt and black pepper.
- 1 tsp. lime juice

Directions:
1. Arrange the cucumber slices on a work area, then divide the other ingredients and roll.
2. Arrange all of the rolls on a tray as an appetizer.

Nutritional information:
200 calories | 6 g fat | 3.4 g fiber | 7.6 g carbs | 3.5 g protein

54. Stuffed Tomatoes with Olives and Cheese

24 servings | Time to prepare: 10 minutes | Time to cook: 0 minutes

Ingredients:
- 2/4 cherry tomatoes, tops removed and insides scooped
- 2 tbsp of olive oil
- 1/4 tsp red pepper flakes
- 1/2 cup crumbled feta cheese
- 2 tbsp. black olive paste
- 1/4 cup torn mint

Directions:
1. In a mixing bowl, combine the olive paste with the other ingredients (excluding the cherry tomatoes) and whisk thoroughly. Stuff the cherry tomatoes with this mixture, then place them on a dish as an appetizer.

Nutritional information:
136 calories | 8.6 g fat | 4.8 g fiber | 5.6 g carbs | 5.1 g protein

55. *Chili Mango and Watermelon Salsa*

12 servings | Time to prepare: 5 minutes | Time to cook: 0 minutes

Ingredients:
- 1 chopped red tomato
- To taste, season with salt and black pepper.
- 1 cup seedless watermelon, peeled and cubed
- 1 sliced red onion
- 2 peeled and cut mangos
- 1/4 cup cilantro, chopped
- 2 chile peppers, chopped
- 3 tablespoons lime juice
- Pita chips to serve

Directions:
1. Toss the tomato, watermelon, onion, and other ingredients (except the pita chips) in a mixing dish. Serve the mixture in tiny cups with pita chips on the side.

Nutritional information:
62 calories | 1.3 g fiber | 3.9 g carbohydrates | 2.3 g protein

56. *Avocado Dip*

8 servings | Time to prepare: 5 minutes | Time to cook: 0 minutes

Ingredients:
- 12 c. thick cream
- 1 chopped green chili pepper

- Season with salt and pepper to taste.
- 4 pitted, peeled, and chopped avocados
- 1/4 cup lime juice
- 1 cup chopped cilantro

Directions:

1. Blend the cream, avocados, and other ingredients in a blender until smooth. Divide the mixture into serving dishes and serve chilled as a party dip.

Nutritional information:

200 calories | 14.5 g fat | 3.8 g fiber | 8.1 g carbs | 7.6 g protein

57. Goat Cheese and Chives Spread

4 servings | Time to prepare: 10 minutes |Time to cook: 0 minutes

Ingredients:

- 2 ounces crumbled goat cheese
- 3/4 cup sour cream
- 2 teaspoons chopped chives
- 1 teaspoon of lemon juice
- To taste, season with salt and black pepper.
- 2 tbsp extra-virgin olive oil

Directions:

1. In a mixing bowl, combine the goat cheese, cream, and other ingredients and stir well. Refrigerate for 10 minutes before serving as a party spread.

Nutritional information:

220 calories | 11.5 g fat | 4.8 g fiber | 8.9 g carbs | 5.6 g protein

58. Dip with Creamy Spinach and Shallots

4 servings | Time to prepare: 10 minutes | Time to cook: 0 minutes

Ingredients:
- 1 pound spinach, coarsely chopped
- 2 shallots, chopped
- 2 tablespoons mint, chopped
- 3/4 cup soft cream cheese
- To taste, season with salt and black pepper.

Directions:
1. In a blender, add the spinach, shallots, and other ingredients, and pulse until smooth. Divide the mixture into small bowls and serve as a party dip.

Nutritional information:
204 calories | 11.5 g fat | 3.1 g fiber | 4.2 g carbs| 5.9 g protein

59. Artichoke Feta Dip

8 servings | Time to prepare: 10 minutes | Time to cook: 30 minutes

Ingredients:
- 8 ounces artichoke hearts, drained and quartered
- 3/4 cup basil, chopped
- 3/4 cup green olives, pitted and chopped
- 1 cup parmesan cheese, grated
- 5 ounces crumbled feta cheese

Directions:
1. In a food processor, combine the artichokes, basil, and other ingredients, pulse well, and transfer to a baking dish.
2. Place in the oven for 30 minutes at 375° F and serve as a party dip.

Nutritional information:
186 calories | 12.4 g fat | 0.9 g fiber | 2.6 g carbs | 1.5 g protein

60. Wrapped Plums

8 servings |Time to prepare: 5 minutes | Time to cook: 0 minutes

Ingredients:
- 2 ounces of prosciutto, sliced into 16 pieces
- 4 plums, quartered
- 1 tablespoon chopped chives
- a pinch of crushed red pepper flakes

Directions:
1. Wrap each plum quarter in a prosciutto slice, put on a dish, sprinkle with chives and pepper flakes, and serve.

Nutritional information
Calories 30 | Fat 1 g | Fiber 0 g | Carbohydrates 4 g | Protein 2 g

61. Sandwich Bites with Cucumber

12 servings | Time to prepare: 5 minutes | Time to cook: 0 minutes

Ingredients:
- 1 cucumber, thinly sliced
- 8 slices whole wheat bread
- 2 tbsp softened cream cheese
- 1 tablespoon chopped chives
- 1/4 cup peeled, pitted, and mashed avocado
- 1 teaspoon dijon mustard
- To taste, season with salt and black pepper.

Directions:
1. Spread the mashed avocado on each bread slice, then top with the other ingredients except the cucumber slices. Divide the cucumber slices among the bread pieces, cut each slice in thirds, and serve as an appetizer.

Nutritional information
Calories: 187 | fat: 12.4 g | fiber: 2.1 g | carbs: 4.5 g | protein: 8.2 g

62. *Vegetable Fritters*

8 servings | Time to prepare: 10 minutes | Time to cook: 10 minutes

Ingredients:
- 2 minced garlic cloves
- 2 yellow onions minced,
- 4 scallions sliced,
- 2 carrots diced,
- 2 teaspoons cumin grated,
- 1/2 teaspoon turmeric powder powdered
- To taste, season with salt and black pepper.
- 1/4 teaspoon coriander, crushed
- 2 tablespoons chopped parsley
- 1/4 teaspoon lemon juice
- 1/2 c. almond flour
- 2 peeled and shredded beets
- 2 whisked eggs
- 1/4 cup tapioca starch
- three tbsp olive oil

Directions:
1. In a mixing bowl, combine the garlic, onions, scallions, and the other ingredients (excluding the oil), stir well, and create medium fritters out of this mixture.
2. Heat the oil in a pan over medium-high heat, then add the fritters and cook for 5 minutes on each side before serving.

Nutritional information:
Calories 209 | Fat 11.2 g | Fiber 3 g | Carbohydrates 4.4 g | Protein 4.8 g

PART 3

10 SUCCESSFUL TIPS FOR A SUSTAINABLE MEDITERRANEAN DASH DIET JOURNEY

Embarking on a Mediterranean DASH (Dietary Approaches to Stop Hypertension) journey can be an enriching experience, promoting not just a healthier lifestyle but also a deeper connection with food and well-being. This fusion of the heart-healthy Mediterranean diet with the science-backed DASH principles emphasizes the consumption of whole, unprocessed foods while reducing the intake of sodium and unhealthy fats. To make your Mediterranean DASH diet journey not only successful but also sustainable, consider the following 10 tips:

1. Emphasize Fresh and Seasonal Produce

Variety is key: Incorporate a diverse array of fruits and vegetables into your meals, aiming for a rich spectrum of colors. Opt for seasonal produce whenever possible, as they are at their peak flavor and nutritional value.

2. Prioritize Whole Grains and Legumes

Opt for whole grains: Replace refined grains with whole grain options like quinoa, brown rice, and whole wheat. Additionally, include legumes such as lentils, chickpeas, and beans, which are excellent sources of fiber and plant-based protein.

3. Include a Variety of Healthy Fats

Favor healthy fats: Utilize sources like extra virgin olive oil, nuts, seeds, and avocados, which are rich in monounsaturated and polyunsaturated fats, promoting heart health and overall well-being.

4. Reduce Added Sugars and Processed Foods

Minimize processed foods: Limit your intake of processed and packaged foods, which often contain high levels of added sugars, unhealthy fats, and preservatives. Instead, opt for whole, natural foods to support your health goals.

5. Experiment with Herbs and Spices for Flavor

Elevate flavors naturally: Use a wide variety of herbs and spices like basil, oregano, thyme, and rosemary to enhance the taste of your dishes without relying on excessive salt or sugar.

6. Incorporate Fish and Poultry Regularly

Include lean protein sources: Integrate fish, especially those rich in omega-3 fatty acids like salmon, mackerel, and sardines, into your weekly meal plan. Incorporate lean poultry like chicken and turkey as alternative protein sources.

7. Practice Mindful Eating and Portion Control

Be mindful of your meals: Focus on savoring each bite and paying attention to your body's hunger and fullness cues. Portion control plays a crucial role in maintaining a healthy weight and preventing overeating.

8. Stay Hydrated with Water and Herbal Teas

Hydration is key: Aim to drink an adequate amount of water throughout the day. Opt for herbal teas as a flavorful and hydrating alternative, steering clear of sugary beverages and excessive caffeine.

9. Engage in Regular Physical Activity

Prioritize movement: Incorporate regular physical activity into your daily routine, whether it's a brisk walk, a yoga session, or any other form of exercise that brings you joy and keeps you active.

10. Foster a Supportive and Positive Food Environment

Cultivate a healthy food environment: Surround yourself with a supportive community that shares similar dietary goals and values. Create an environment at home that encourages and reinforces your commitment to a sustainable Mediterranean DASH diet.

Adhering to these tips can help you maintain a balanced and sustainable Mediterranean DASH diet journey, fostering a sense of well-being, vitality, and overall health that lasts a lifetime.

CONCLUSION AND LONG-TERM BENEFITS OF THE MEDITERRANEAN DASH DIET

In the pursuit of sustainable and enjoyable approaches to healthy eating, the Mediterranean DASH diet stands as a beacon of culinary delight and nutritional balance. This harmonious fusion of the time-honored Mediterranean diet and the scientifically-backed DASH (Dietary Approaches to Stop Hypertension) principles transcends mere dietary restrictions; it embodies a lifestyle of profound nourishment, wellness, and joy. By incorporating the rich tapestry of flavors, textures, and nutrients inherent in this diet, individuals can experience a transformative journey toward improved overall well-being.

A Sustainable Approach to Healthy Eating:

The Mediterranean DASH diet advocates for the consumption of whole, unprocessed foods, highlighting the importance of sourcing locally grown produce and incorporating seasonal ingredients. By fostering a connection to the earth and its natural bounty, this dietary approach not only benefits personal health but also supports sustainable agricultural practices and local communities. Through mindful food choices and an emphasis on plant-based foods, the Mediterranean DASH diet promotes a sustainable food system that nurtures both the body and the planet.

An Enjoyable Culinary Experience:

Embracing the Mediterranean DASH diet unlocks a world of culinary exploration, where vibrant flavors, aromatic herbs, and wholesome ingredients come together to create an exquisite tapestry of taste sensations. With a focus on incorporating an abundance of fresh fruits, vegetables, whole grains, lean proteins, and heart-healthy fats, this diet encourages the creation of nourishing and delectable meals that tantalize the taste buds and elevate the dining experience. By indulging in the pleasures of cooking and savoring each bite mindfully, individuals can cultivate a profound appreciation for the art of nourishing the body and soul through food.

The Long-lasting Impact on Overall Well-being:

Beyond the immediate benefits of improved cardiovascular health and blood pressure regulation, the Mediterranean DASH diet fosters a holistic approach to well-being, influencing various facets of life. By adopting this dietary lifestyle, individuals often witness enhanced cognitive function, increased energy levels, and a strengthened immune system. Moreover, the diet's emphasis on whole foods and nutrient-dense ingredients contributes to weight management, fostering a healthy body composition and promoting a positive body image. This holistic approach to well-being extends beyond physical health, as the Mediterranean DASH diet has been shown to contribute to a sense of mental clarity, emotional balance, and overall life satisfaction.

In conclusion, the Mediterranean DASH diet transcends the limitations of a mere dietary regimen, encapsulating a holistic philosophy that nourishes the body, mind, and spirit. By embracing the sustainable and enjoyable culinary practices advocated by this diet, individuals can embark on a transformative journey toward long-term well-being, cultivating a profound connection to food, community, and the fundamental essence of a healthy, fulfilling life.

20 Simple Daily Exercises

The Mediterranean DASH diet emphasizes a combination of nutritious foods and regular physical activity for overall well-being. Here are 20 exercises that complement this dietary approach:

1. Brisk Walking: Enjoy a daily walk in nature or around your neighborhood.

2. Jogging: Incorporate moderate jogging sessions to elevate your heart rate.

3. Swimming: Take a refreshing dip in the pool or the ocean for a full-body workout.

4. Cycling: Explore the outdoors on a bike ride to improve cardiovascular health.

5. Hiking: Connect with nature while challenging your body on scenic trails.

6. Yoga: Practice gentle or dynamic yoga sequences to promote flexibility and mindfulness.

7. Pilates: Strengthen your core and improve posture through targeted Pilates exercises.

8. Dancing: Join a dance class or dance at home to enhance cardiovascular health and mood.

9. Tennis: Enjoy a friendly match of tennis to improve agility and coordination.

10. Aerobic Classes: Participate in aerobic workouts to increase endurance and burn calories.

11. Bodyweight Exercises: Engage in push-ups, squats, lunges, and planks for strength training.

12. Resistance Band Workouts: Use resistance bands to tone muscles and improve flexibility.

13. Stair Climbing: Incorporate climbing stairs to boost leg strength and cardiovascular fitness.

14. Kayaking: Enjoy an upper body workout while exploring waterways and lakes.

15. Rowing: Engage in rowing exercises to improve strength and cardiovascular endurance.

16. Tai Chi: Practice the graceful movements of Tai Chi for improved balance and relaxation.

17. Golf: Engage in a game of golf to enhance focus and promote light physical activity.

18. Zumba: Join a lively Zumba class for an energetic and fun-filled workout.

19. Functional Training: Incorporate exercises that mimic everyday movements for improved functionality.

20. Circuit Training: Combine various exercises in a high-intensity circuit to improve overall fitness levels.

Remember to consult a healthcare professional before starting any new exercise regimen, particularly if you have any preexisting health conditions.

Incorporating a variety of these exercises into your routine can help you maintain a healthy lifestyle that complements the Mediterranean DASH diet, promoting overall well-being and vitality.

28-DAYS MEAL PLAN

Feel free to adjust the meal plan based on your preferences and dietary requirements. Remember to stay hydrated, incorporate healthy snacks, and savor the delicious and nutritious meals that the Mediterranean DASH diet offers. Enjoy this wholesome and flavorful journey!

WEEK 1 MEAL PLAN

MONDAY

BREAKFAST Sweet Potatoes with Coconut Flakes

LUNCH Tuna Salad

SNACKS Meatballs Platters

DINNER Goat Cheese with Fold-Overs

TUESDAY

BREAKFAST French Toast with Applesauce

LUNCH Salad with Salmon

SNACKS Bruschetta with Tomatoes

DINNER Coconut soup for Dinner

WEDNESDAY

BREAKFAST Baking Powder Biscuits

LUNCH Turkey and Mozzarella Sandwich

SNACKS Red Pepper Tapenade

DINNER Tacos de Mariscos (Fish Tacos)

THURSDAY

BREAKFAST Banana and Cinnamon Oatmeal

LUNCH Veggie Soup

SNACKS Salsa de Chili Mango y Watermelon

DINNER Clam chowder

FRIDAY

BREAKFAST Oatmeal Banana Pancakes with Walnuts

LUNCH Salad with Shrimps

SNACKS Eggplant Dip

DINNER Cobb salad

SATURDAY

BREAKFAST Mediterranean toast

LUNCH Spaghetti Squash with Sauce

SNACKS Hummus with Red Peppers

DINNER carbonara

SUNDAY

BREAKFAST Avocado Cup with Egg

LUNCH Lunch salad with quinoa and spinach

SNACKS cucumber bites

DINNER Seeded Cauliflower Soup

NOTES

WEEK 2 MEAL PLAN

MONDAY

BREAKFAST Buckwheat Pancakes with Vanilla Almond Milk

LUNCH Tacos de Pollo (Chicken Tacos)

SNACKS Chili Mango and Watermelon Salsa

DINNER Stuffed bell peppers

TUESDAY

BREAKFAST Muesli Scones

LUNCH Chinese chicken

SNACKS Stuffed Tomatoes with Olives and Cheese

DINNER Asparagus Wrapped in Prosciutto

WEDNESDAY

BREAKFAST Mushroom Spinach Omelet

LUNCH Instant Pot Beef Gyros

SNACKS Avocado Dips

DINNER Zucchini Bars

THURSDAY

BREAKFAST Sweet Potato Waffles

LUNCH Pasta with Meat Sauce

SNACKS Goat Cheese and Chives Spread

DINNER Merjimek (Lentil Soup)

FRIDAY

BREAKFAST Faux Breakfast Hash Brown Cups

LUNCH Instant Pot Egg Sandwiches

SNACKS Artichoke Feta Dip

DINNER Meatball soup

SATURDAY

BREAKFAST Sweet Corn Muffins

LUNCH Pasta with Tuscan chicken

SNACKS Dip with Creamy Spinach and Shallots

DINNER Chicken leak soup

SUNDAY

BREAKFAST Tomato Bruschetta with Basil

LUNCH Teriyaki chicken

SNACKS Wrapped plums

DINNER Egg plant soup

NOTES

WEEK 3 MEAL PLAN

MONDAY

BREAKFAST Oatmeal Banana Pancakes with Walnuts

LUNCH Veggie soup

SNACKS Cucumber Bites

DINNER Seeded Cauliflower Soup

TUESDAY

BREAKFAST Mediterranean Toast

LUNCH Salad and shrimps

SNACKS Egg plant dip

DINNER Cobb salad

WEDNESDAY

BREAKFAST Avocado Cup with Egg

LUNCH Tuna salad

SNACKS Meatballs platters

DINNER Goat cheese with fold-overs

THURSDAY

BREAKFAST Mushroom spinach omelette

LUNCH Tacos de Pollo (Chicken Tacos)

SNACKS Chili Mango and Watermelon Salsa

DINNER Stuffed bell peppers

FRIDAY

BREAKFAST Buckwheat Pancakes with Vanilla Almond Milk

LUNCH Salad with salmon

SNACKS Bruschetta with Tomatoes

DINNER coconut soup

SATURDAY

BREAKFAST muesli scones

LUNCH Turkey and Mozzarella Sandwich

SNACKS Red pepper Tapenade

DINNER Tacos de Mariscos (Fish Tacos)

SUNDAY

BREAKFAST Sweet potatoes waffles

LUNCH Spaghetti Squash with Sauce

SNACKS Hummus with Red Peppers

DINNER Carbonara

NOTES

WEEK 4 MEAL PLAN

MONDAY

BREAKFAST Faux Breakfast Hash Brown Cups

LUNCH Instant pot beef gyros

SNACKS Avocado dips

DINNER Zucchini Bars

TUESDAY

BREAKFAST Sweet corn muffins

LUNCH Pasta with Meat Sauce

SNACKS Goat Cheese and Chives Spread

DINNER Merjimek

WEDNESDAY

BREAKFAST Tomato Bruschetta with Basil

LUNCH Teriyaki chicken

SNACKS wrapped plums

DINNER Egg plant soup

THURSDAY

BREAKFAST Oatmeal Banana Pancakes with Walnuts

LUNCH Veggie soup

SNACKS Cucumber Bites

DINNER Seeded Cauliflower Soup

FRIDAY

BREAKFAST Mediterranean Toast

LUNCH Salad with shrimps

SNACKS Egg plant dips

DINNER Cobb salad

SATURDAY

BREAKFAST Avocado Cup with Egg

LUNCH Tuna salad

SNACKS meatballs platters

DINNER Goat Cheese with Fold-Overs

SUNDAY

BREAKFAST Mushroom Spinach Omelet

LUNCH Tacos de Pollo (Chicken Tacos)

SNACKS Chili Mango and Watermelon Salsa

DINNER Stuffed Bell Peppers

NOTES